The Telehealth OT

A guide to teach occupational therapists about telehealth

DR. REINA M. OLIVERA

Copyright © 2020 Dr. Reina M. Olivera

All rights reserved.

ISBN: 9798619429688

DEDICATION

This book is for the techie-at-heart and for the millennial that grew up on an iPhone or Android. It is even for the baby boomers that have been treating for 30+ years, but just need a change. It is for the introverts that don't ever want to leave the house to go to the holiday party. It is for the military spouse that moves around a lot and is tired of job applications and interview after interview. Most of all, it is for the new mom that needs the flexibility to take care of her baby while still putting that degree to good use. Telehealth is for occupational therapists all over the world that aspire to move with the changing times and keep up with what the future holds.

CONTENTS

	Acknowledgments	i
	Disclaimer	ii
1	Introduction to Telehealth	1
2	Benefits and Concerns for Telehealth Practice	13
3	Telehealth as a Service Delivery Model	19
4	Laws and Regulations	29
5	Employment	39
6	Referrals and Payment Source	45

ACKNOWLEDGMENTS

First and foremost, I would like to acknowledge my family. My amazing husband who has been extremely supportive and patient through this entire process. You have always said, "No quiero ser una piedra en tu camino" and for that, I thank you.

My two beautiful daughters, you are my "why". I want to show you what it means to be a successful woman in this crazy world you are growing in. My mom, thank you for your help with editing this book. I appreciate you.

Next, I want to take this opportunity to thank a few individuals that have been willing to help me on my telehealth journey. Tracy Davis, you were the only occupational therapist that let me observe your sessions when I was in school learning about telehealth. I'm forever grateful for your teamwork spirit. You are truly an asset to the telehealth world! To Jana Cason, I idolized you before I even had the chance to speak to you. The papers you wrote for the occupational therapy community are extremely valuable and were my introduction to telehealth. You continue to open the doors to more telehealth opportunities for me. To my telehealth capstone and faculty mentors, Dr. Evelyn Terrell and Dr. Sandra Dunbar. You both taught me so much through the doctoral program and really pushed me past my comfort zone for optimal learning experiences. I hope this book makes you proud.

DISCLAIMER

This is a guide including information that I have gathered over years on telehealth practice within the field of occupational therapy. The information in this book is not meant to serve as legal advice. Please be sure to consult with a business telehealth attorney prior to beginning telehealth work, especially if you're considering opening a private telehealth practice. Although I have made every effort to ensure that the information in this book was correct at press time, I do not assume and hereby disclaim any liability to any party for any loss, damage, or disruption caused by errors or omissions, whether such errors or omissions result from negligence, accident, or any other cause.

1 INTRODUCTION TO TELEHEALTH

Telehealth is the use of telecommunication to deliver health care. Often times, in the world of occupational and physical therapists it is referred to as telerehabilitation or teletherapy, in the world of speech and language pathologists it is referred to as telepractice, among physicians it is referred to as telemedicine, and in general healthcare settings it is referred to as telecare and e-health. Sometimes these terms are used interchangeably, but I have found that the term telehealth is the most common in our profession; as it does not narrow the practice to a rehabilitative model of treatment.

Types of Telehealth

Telehealth can be divided into two main types: synchronous

and asynchronous. These are just fancy words meaning that the communication is either happening between two people at the same time, or one person has created something that the other is viewing at a later time.

Let's start with asynchronous, because it is probably the least heard of. Asynchronous telehealth is also called store-and-forward. Just as the name implies, some kind of media is being captured and stored. It is then sent (forwarded) to someone else to view it. For example, an x-ray can be taken at one location, stored in a medical database, and sent to a radiologist at another location for viewing and diagnosing. In occupational therapy, this technology is being used to send clients home exercise programs, in the forms of video and pictures, for the client to use independently. Similarly, the client can take a video of their progress and send it to the occupational therapist for feedback.

Now let's talk about synchronous communication. Synchronous telehealth can be accomplished via phone or video calls. Video conferencing is similar to the use of FaceTime to call a friend or family member. Unlike asynchronous communication, these calls are live and interactive. Video calls are the most common form of telehealth; therefore, that is what I will be referring to for the remainder of the book.

Technology

What do you need to implement a telehealth session?

First and foremost, you and your client need a device. This device can be a computer, laptop, tablet, or phone. The device must have a camera that is either built-in or connected externally through the USB port. Some practitioners have taken this a step further and use both, the built-in camera and an external one that is pointed at the table surface. The client can be setup with an external camera (Figure 1), so the occupational therapist can see what the child is doing (i.e. Handwriting). The device being used must also include an audio feature with both input and output. Again, this can be built-in or installed externally. Some occupational therapists choose to use a headset (Figure 2) for patient privacy and better sound quality.

Figure 1   Figure 2

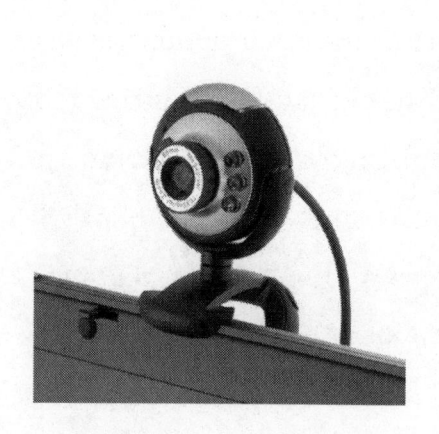

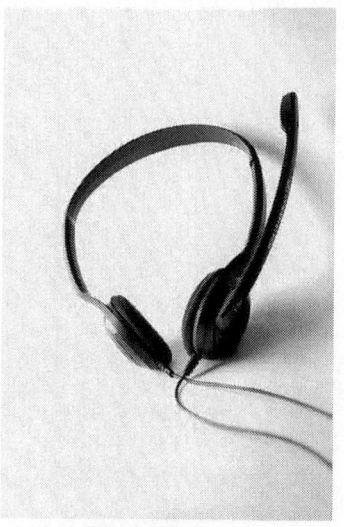

These devices need to be connected to a reliable Internet connection. The recommended bandwidth speed is at least 15 megabits per second for downloads and 5 megabits per second for uploads. You can go to speedtest.net to check your Internet speed. One recommendation for troubleshooting connectivity issues is to use a wired Internet connection instead of Wi-Fi, by plugging directly into the router or modem with an Ethernet cable. For patients wanting to use their mobile network, it is a good idea to advise them that streaming video uses a good amount of data.

Now, let's talk about the software. Video sessions occur over a secure platform. Some are as simple as a regular video call similar to FaceTime (please note that FaceTime is not HIPAA compliant…we'll go over that in a little bit) and other platforms include other options, such as screen sharing and apps that the client can use during the session. Some of the better-known companies that are offering telehealth platforms are Simple Practice, Blink Session, TheraPlatform, TheraNest, Zoom, Doxy.me, and VSee. As of the writing of this book, Simple Practice offers a very simple video chat feature with screen share technology. In comparison, TheraPlatform and Blink Session incorporate fun apps that a client can play to work on different goals setup by the therapist.

Simple Practice, TheraNest, Blink Session, and TheraPlatform are all-inclusive platforms that have billing, scheduling, and documentation. All three have a virtual waiting room, so that the clients aren't going into each other's video sessions. Blink Session has a very unique "group sessions" feature with an unlimited number of guests. This enables collaboration between the client, family, and multiple providers, if needed. Blink Session has a digital dry-erase board that both the client and the therapist can use. They also have a library of resources available for therapists to use in each session, which includes flash cards, PDF documents, videos, and more. Blink Session is one of the only platforms that give the ability to record sessions and store them in their cloud, eliminating the need to store videos on your computer. Storing videos in their cloud also makes it super simple to retrieve them during the session for future use. Blink Session has three pricing plans: basic, standard, and advanced, starting at $38, $64, and $76 per month for 1 staff user, and increases based on the number of users.

Some of the features unique to TheraPlatform include the built-in apps and games (available on the Pro Plus version only), an in-session documentation option, and secure in-session chat. Like Blink Session, TheraPlatform also has a digital dry-erase board, group sessions, and screen sharing. TheraPlatform's basic plan is $29 per month for a single provider. Their pro plan is $39 per month for the first provider and $29 for each additional provider. The pro plus plan starts at $59 per month and $39 for each additional provider. Please note that each plan includes certain features. For details, please see the Pricing Plans section on their website (https://www.theraplatform.com/Pricing).

Simple Practice has two options for the solo practitioner including the essential plan, which is $39 per month, and the professional plan, which is $59 per month. With the professional plan, you can add an unlimited number of clinicians for $39 per month each. For both the essential and the professional plan, you will need to add $10 per therapist, per month, for the telehealth feature. Until recently, the telehealth feature was a simple two-way camera made just for video chatting. Now, Simple Practice has added a screen sharing feature, which practitioners are very happy about. Another great feature is the paperless client intakes. These forms are customizable and are sent to the client before their first appointment; thereby, cutting back on paperwork time during the initial evaluation.

In my opinion, the platform that is most comparable to Simple Practice is TheraNest. The key difference is that TheraNest bills per number of active clients beginning at $38 per month for up to 30 active clients, instead of billing per user. They have the same $10 per therapist, per month, fee for telehealth. The telehealth option is also a simple video chat with group and screen share features. TheraNest may be a good option for those practitioners starting a solo-practice who are not necessarily looking to grow too big.

Now let's talk about Zoom, Doxy.me, and VSee. These are video platforms and do not include billing or documentation. Zoom is probably one of the most popular video conferencing software programs in the market. It is pretty basic in that it is mostly used for video chats, but some other features include a digital dry-erase board, screen sharing, recording, and scheduling. The only downside about Zoom is that the free version is not HIPAA compliant, forcing healthcare professionals to pay a hefty $200 per month for the HIPAA compliant version.

On the other hand, both Doxy.me and VSee have HIPAA compliant versions that are free. VSee is more of a medical application, however, if you're just looking for a video platform, it can be a great option. Doxy.me is another great option for a video platform. Doxy.me always promises to keep a free version, as they believe that cost should not be a barrier to telemedicine. The great thing about Doxy.me is that there is no download required. They simply provide the client with a link to click on right from the browser. Like some of the other platforms mentioned above, Doxy.me has a waiting room and a chat feature. They also have a professional version for $35 per month for an individual and a clinic version starting at $50 per month and increases depending on the number of providers. VSee also has a plus version for individuals for $49 per month and a standard and an advanced version for practices at $199 and $499 per month, per provider, respectively.

Patient Privacy and Security

Up next is probably one of the most concerning topics in the healthcare field...HIPAA. Please make note, that it is H-I-P-A-A as in Health Insurance Portability and Accountability Act not H-I-P-P-A, as in "too close to the word hippo". I've seen way too many professionals spell this incorrectly, so I hope that now you will always remember that this privacy act is for human beings and not hippopotami. I will get off my soapbox, now.

I want to clear up a huge misconception regarding cash-based private practice telehealth. Some people are under the impression that HIPAA does not apply to them if they do not take insurance. The privacy act is for the protection and security of patient's medical information. This law is in place whether or not the client uses insurance to pay for services.

Here are some tips to make sure you remain HIPAA compliant:

- Always keep notes and documents locked (in the telehealth world, this means using a password on your computer and always logging off any programs containing patient information)
- Make sure that no one can hear patient

information (I suggest using a headset during video calls to avoid others hearing what the client is saying)
- In private practice, be sure to have a Business Associate Agreement with any companies you use (including email provider, phone, electronic medical record software, and telehealth software)
- When communicating via email, confirm the patient's email address prior to sending medical information; understand that the patient has the right to request communication via alternative means
- It is best practice to have the patient's written consent for treatment via telehealth (include potential risks/benefits, options for technology failure, and their rights to stop treatment)

Practice Settings

Before I go on to discuss the benefits and potential concerns for telehealth in occupational therapy, I will briefly mention the settings that telehealth is being used in. If you have already started to look for information on telehealth, be it while looking for a job opportunity or thinking about setting out into private practice, you probably already noticed that pediatrics dominates this technological area of practice. That said, there are many occupational therapists in the adult world that are venturing out into telehealth as well.

In pediatrics, telehealth is being used in schools, home-based, and out in the community. Researchers (Little, Pope, Wallisch, and Dunn, 2018) used telehealth to implement a parent-coaching model for children with autism. They found that the use of telehealth increased parent efficacy and child participation. Via telehealth and with the assistance of the occupational therapist, parents were able to formulate and reach goals to improve the child's adaptive behaviors in the home and community environments. Home-based telehealth often serves as a supplement to school-based services, which are, likely, only addressing educational goals.

In adults, telehealth is being used in acute care within the hospital setting, in rehabilitation facilities, including both inpatient and outpatient, in homes, and in the community. The Veterans Health Administration (Gately, Trudeau, and Moo, 2020) has used telehealth in assisting caregivers of patients with dementia to complete home-safety evaluations. Here, the caregivers were instructed to navigate the home while holding a laptop or tablet. The practitioner then observed the home environment and gave recommendations such as lighting, flooring, counters, etc.

There are also specific diagnosis-based telehealth programs, such as Un*limb*ited Wellness, a telehealth program for adults with upper limb difference. This program offers access to peers and information on strategies to prevent overuse injuries, social isolation, and improve advocacy skills with medical providers.

Another interesting study (Cotton, Russell, Johnston, and Legge, 2017) used telehealth technology to train therapists to perform a pre-employment functional assessment. They found no statistically significant difference in therapists who were trained in-person versus those trained via video conferencing and those trained by asynchronous video modules. As I previously mentioned, telehealth also includes the use of video technology in healthcare education and this study is a great example of that.

2 BENEFITS AND CONCERNS FOR TELEHEALTH PRACTICE

Benefits for the Client

There are many benefits to using telehealth from the client perspective. If you have done any research in this area, you will notice that telehealth originally started for individuals living in rural communities to have access to healthcare. In a world where technology is the way of the future, it makes the most sense that if someone lives an hour from the closest provider, that they are better off connecting with them via video conferencing. The only issue that I have personally come across in this scenario is that the client has "spotty" cell phone service. Therefore, it's very important that you run through the setup process with the client, ensuring that the Internet speed is adequate (see Chapter 1 for the technology details).

In this next section, I'm going to tell you a story:

A mom of a child with autism spectrum disorder goes through the struggle of getting her son in the car and driving to the clinic. Despite the tantrums and meltdowns that her child had before it was time to leave, she *hates* being late and gets to the clinic 15 minutes before her son's appointment time. They already know the check-in process, so she writes her son's name on the clipboard and proceeds to sit in the waiting room. By the way, she couldn't find childcare for her daughter, so she's in the waiting room now, too. The 15 minutes in the waiting room are pure chaos, there are children running around everywhere and exactly at 3 o'clock all the therapists come out to tell other parents about their child's progress. Yes, in the waiting room, because the parents at this clinic are accustomed to using therapy time as respite. Regardless, when it's this mom's turn to speak to the occupational therapist about her son, she can't even bring herself to focus. She is so overwhelmed and says, "If the sensory input here bothers me, I can't imagine what my son is feeling." When she realizes this, she begins looking for a telehealth option. That is when she found my services and, believe it or not, she was practically in tears when she heard about my business model. She's been looking for an option where she didn't have to live in the waiting room and miss everything that was happening with her son during therapy time.

This is based on a true story. One of the benefits of telehealth is eliminating the waiting room experience. Additionally, it provides occupational therapists the opportunity to provide interventions in the child's natural environment. Another benefit is the ability to involve family members, who are not in the same location, via group calls. Lastly, another huge benefit of telehealth is for the child that is immunocompromised. Telehealth eliminates the need for the child to be exposed to illnesses, by allowing them to stay in their home environment to receive services.

Benefits for the Practitioner

There are also many benefits from the practitioner viewpoint. As I mentioned in the introduction, many occupational therapists interested in telehealth are new moms, because one of the biggest benefits is working from home. I speak from experience when I say that it's extremely hard to leave your 3 month old (the expectation in the United States of America) to go back to work. Therefore, having a work-from-home option becomes a new happy medium where a new mom can stay home with her baby while setting aside some time for seeing clients via video. Aside from working from home, occupational therapists are able to "play" with time zones. If they are located in Eastern Time Zone and want to work at night, after the kids go to bed, they can work with families that are in Pacific Time Zone that may just be getting home from work. Another benefit from an occupational therapist perspective is increased client outcomes. This is due to a few reasons, including decreased cancellations and increased parent carryover. How many of you, who work in an outpatient clinic right now, have cancellations the minute a drop of rain falls from the sky? Rain = going home from work early; and in some private clinics, cancellations = no pay. Speaking of private practice, if you decide that you want to start your own telehealth business, another benefit is that there are minimal overhead costs. Don't get me wrong, it's not as affordable to start a telehealth business as you might think, but it goes without saying that you don't have to pay for rent and incur other monthly fees that come with a brick and mortar location.

Concerns

When I give presentations on telehealth, there are always a few "old school" therapists that feel they just can't get away from having their hands on the child. These are the occupational therapists that are Neuro-Developmental Treatment (NDT) certified and grew up with that physical touch. This is one of the concerns about using telehealth as a service delivery model. You have to accept the fact that you will no longer be touching people unless you are involved in some type of hybrid model, where telehealth is a supplement to in-person sessions. Another concern is that it's not *whether* technology fails it's *when* technology fails. As with our phones, televisions, radios, cars, and all other electronics, the telehealth software, Internet, and devices are bound to fail at one point or another. However, as occupational therapists we are trained to be flexible and to adapt, so having a backup plan is a quick solution to that. Some options are to have a secondary telehealth platform, to do a phone call, or, as a last resort, you can always reschedule. The last concern for working in telehealth is the state licensure laws. As of the writing of this book, the predominating rule is that you must be licensed where your client resides. Some states take this a step further and require the practitioner physically be located in the same state as the client, meaning you can't go on vacation in another country and continue seeing your clients. There are some states that have very specific telehealth laws. Laws and regulations will be discussed in Chapter 4, but please refer to https://www.cchpca.org for the most up-to-date information.

3 TELEHEALTH AS A SERVICE DELIVERY MODEL

The very first thing that I learned about telehealth is that it is a service delivery model. What does this mean? It means that we are using the same critical reasoning skills to evaluate, plan, and treat, as in any other setting. There are some key differences and helpful tips included in this chapter.

Documentation

Writing a note for telehealth is basically the same as writing one for any other setting, with the exception that some states require a phrase that says that the services were provided via telehealth. Please check your particular state laws and regulations, as they are all very different. In general, documentation should include evaluation, goals, a narrative or S.O.A.P. note, as applicable, progress notes, and a discharge note. The goals should not be about telehealth, but rather about participation in the child's occupations. For example, it should not be, "Child will attend to video call for 5 minutes with minimal verbal cues." It should be, "Child will attend to 5 minutes of dressing task with minimal verbal cues."

    Another consideration for documentation is what application or software to use. Documentation styles range from use of pen and paper, to the use of technological advances, and to the use of specific programs. There are many telehealth platforms that include documentation features. There are also a variety of software programs that are specifically for electronic medical record (EMR) charting. I will not be going over those software programs, but there is ClinicSource, Nota.app (specifically for occupational therapist and speech language pathologists), Jane.app, and Fusion Web Clinic (specifically for pediatrics). Just to name a few.

Evaluation

Although the documentation process is pretty similar to

other settings, the evaluation process can actually be quite different, as you can imagine. First, I'll start by saying that many big assessment tool providers are updating to modern technology and converting some of the popular assessments into digital form. Below are some examples, but please know that this list is not all-inclusive and that more assessment tools will continue to be created as of the publication of this book.

Most of you have heard of Pearson Assessments, right? This includes the Sensory Profile, the Bayley Scales of Infant and Toddler Development Screening Test, the Beery VMI, the Bruininks-Oseretsky Test of Motor Proficiency: Second Edition (BOT-2), the Peabody Developmental Motor Scales, and much more. Pearson has a web-based system called Q-global that is for test administration, scoring, and reporting. Q-global includes over 60 assessments including the Vineland-3, the Bayley-4, the BOT-2, and the Sensory Profile 2. There are many questions that come up about how these assessments can be accomplished online without the in-person interaction. Below is a link to Dr. Winnie Dunn's thoughts on the digital format of the Sensory Profile 2.

https://www.brainshark.com/1/player/en/pearsonassessments?intk=546921588&fb=0&r3f1=&custom=sp2faq1

If you purchased the printed version of this book and this link is way too long to type out, I invite you to go on the Pearson Assessments website and browse the tools along with the FAQs for each one. Briefly, this video explains that when the Sensory Profile was standardized, it was given to parents to fill out without an explanation of each question. Personally, I know that when I have given the Sensory Profile to parents in the clinic, they typically ask questions and we explain what each area is referring to. However, Dr. Dunn explains that the assessment was intended to work without clarification. Whether providing a parent with a paper or digital format, they should be completing the assessment independently. Therefore, giving parents access to the digital format separately from a video call, allows them the time to think about each question and answer to the best of their ability without our assistance.

Another assessment tool provider that you may be familiar with is WPS Publishing. They are the providers of the Adaptive Behavior Assessment System, the Autism Diagnostic Observation Schedule (ADOS), and much more. If you're familiar with ADOS, you know that it requires a lot of objects/toys and, therefore, it is not one that is appropriate for telehealth. WPS Publishing has a digital version of the Sensory Processing Measure (SPM), which is an appropriate tool for telehealth. The SPM is a questionnaire that includes teacher and parent forms. These forms are available in electronic format and WPS Publishing provides an online evaluation system that includes administration, scoring, and reporting of the SPM.

The last assessment tool that I will mention is the Behavior Rating Inventory of Executive Function, Second Edition (BRIEF-2). The BRIEF-2 Digital Kit includes teacher, parent, and self-report forms on PARiConnect, the online assessment platform by PAR, "the leading publisher of psychological assessment materials."

Now that I have your wheels turning about digital assessment tools, let's take a few steps back and mention an alternative. If you have paper forms, you can also opt to mail the client a packet with a paid return envelope. Let's fast forward again…how about emailing the client the PDF format of a non-standardized tool or a developmental checklist? In addition to deciding the method of assessing the child, you will also be completing a parent/caregiver interview as usual. Be sure to include questions about diagnosis, concerns, medical and developmental history, other specialist involved, family members, and all other pertinent information. You will also be conducting client observation to obtain information on behaviors and skills. One of my favorite parts of the telehealth evaluation is the environmental observation, especially if you are doing home-based treatment. Here, I ask the parent to show me the home, playroom, and school space (if applicable). I also ask what supplies or tools they have available that can be used during therapy time. You can also gain information about the school or community environment, accordingly.

Intervention

As I mentioned earlier, the first step to getting into telehealth is accepting the fact that you will not be touching a client. Verbal communication is key. Here are some communication tips that are going to help you have a successful session:

1. Practice giving instructions without physical touch – As occupational therapists, we love people and most of us were trained to use therapeutic touch with our clients. Learning and accepting that treatment via telehealth completely eliminates physical touch is very difficult. However, once

you have committed to video calls, you must learn how to provide instructions with, primarily, verbal cues. You will have the option to use visual cues, such as creating a craft beforehand, so your client sees the final product, or using the screen share technology to show a website or other resource. However, when you want a parent to have their child sit in a particular place or get into a specific position (i.e. prone or quadruped), you must communicate this effectively without physical touch.

2. Practice looking at the camera lens while speaking – Eye contact is just as important in online communication as it is in person. In order for the video call to feel more personal, the client needs to feel like you are looking at them. Avoid looking at yourself on the camera. Instead, practice looking at the camera lens. Some choose to place a picture of an eye or a person right next to the camera lens as a reminder. With some practice, looking at the camera lens will become second nature.

3. Explain the process – This idea of communicating

via video is probably just as new to you as it is to your client. Therefore, it is extremely important that you explain to them what they can expect from you throughout the session.

Practice this in front of a mirror before your first client. After you're done practicing your communication in front of the mirror, it's time to start planning the actual intervention session. There are numerous ways to go about this. It depends on the client and what goals you are working on. Below are some options for telehealth intervention practice.

- Emailing the parent or caregiver a few days or a week prior to the next session. You can send them worksheets to print out, handouts to review, forms to fill out, or a list of supplies to prepare.
- Shipping the family a kit including supplies that you would like the child to use.
- Using apps through the platform of choice, such as TheraPlatform or Blink Session.
- Creating a model of a craft activity that you would like the child to do.
- Preparing an external camera to point at your

work surface for the child to see.
- Using a parent-coaching model, which includes asking probing questions, figuring out the intervention ideas *with* the parents, and providing feedback.

Discharge

As with all practice settings, you must use your expertise to determine when a client has met goals or is displaying a plateau in their progress. Determining the appropriate time to discharge a client is the same in telehealth. However, there are some differences in the process of discharging a telehealth client. It is best practice to provide a digital version of a home exercise program and send a follow up email with final recommendations. Be sure to document the reason for discharge, which goals were or were not met, and the final information provided, including recommendations to other professionals and reasons to seek treatment again in the future.

4 LAWS AND REGULATIONS

This is probably the section of this book that I was dreading the most. Why? Well, because, all the state laws are different. If you haven't heard the great (almost amazing) news yet, our profession will be getting a licensure compact by 2024. What does that mean? It means a little more freedom to practice across state lines. However, there is a caveat. States will be allowed to choose whether or not they participate in the OT Compact. There are also some other considerations, including background checks and application for privileges to practice in other states.

While we sit and wait for politicians to do their thing with the OT Compact, we need to be acquainted with the laws of all 50 states. Keep in mind that some states are stricter than others and some don't even have anything in place. That said, let's cover some of the laws that stand out from the long list of laws and regulations. Please bear in mind that the following information is from Fall 2019. If you are reading this in the future, there are likely new laws already in place, so be sure to do your research. For more information go to The National Telehealth Policy Resource Center website and/or consult with an attorney.

Oh, and please be advised that these laws and regulations are for telehealth in general, including medicine, rehab, mental health, etc. Some states specifically mention occupational therapy, but as with a lot of things, most don't mention it at all. "What is occupational therapy anyway? I don't even have a job anymore. I'm retired." All jokes aside, here are the states that stood out to me.

States that specifically mention occupational therapy:
- California
    - "Informed consent must be obtained by the occupational therapist prior to use of telehealth to deliver services"
- Delaware
    - Includes specific definitions of telehealth and telemedicine as they apply to occupational therapy

- Idaho
    - Lists occupational therapists as eligible providers
- Illinois
    - Includes occupational therapists as those allowed to provide telehealth services as of January 1, 2019
- Kentucky
    - Occupational therapy evaluation and treatment is under "additional covered services in administration regulations"
    - Lists eligible providers not in a Community Mental Health Center that are eligible to provide telehealth services including occupational therapists
    - Occupational therapist must obtain patient consent
- Minnesota
    - Occupational therapists/occupational therapy assistants are listed under "eligible providers"
    - Minnesota Health Care Program will pay for some rehabilitation services (including occupational therapy) via telehealth, as long as the same standards and ethics are held as in

face-to-face
- Includes billing code modifiers and location code to be used
- Limits 3 telehealth sessions per week
- Does not cover materials to be sent to client
- Includes occupational therapy in the list of providers for the Early Intensive Developmental and Behavioral Intervention

- Montana
  - Includes occupational therapists under "eligible providers under parity law"
- Nevada
  - Does not cover telehealth occupational therapy in home health
- New York
  - Lists occupational therapists as eligible providers for home telehealth services
- Texas
  - Defines telehealth as it pertains to occupational therapy and specifies that the occupational therapists licensed in Texas should only provide telehealth to clients located in Texas at the time the services are rendered
- Wyoming

- Defines telehealth as it pertains to occupational therapy

Next, let's review some of the state statutes mentioned in the American Occupational Therapy Association's "Occupational Therapy and Telehealth: State Statutes, Regulations and Regulatory Board Statements" document. This document can be accessed on the AOTA website and is available to members only. Here are some of the state rules that stood out to me:

- Alaska
    - Occupational therapist must be physically present in the state while performing telerehabilitation
    - Businesses practicing telemedicine must register for the Telemedicine Business Registry
- Arkansas
    - Professional relationship must be established with the client and include a history obtained with the provider during the video call, rather than completed by the patient and sent to the provider
    - The laws appear to be geared toward

telemedicine, but, by their definition, a healthcare professional includes anyone who is licensed or certified to provide health care within their profession
- California
  - Telehealth consent must be obtained
  - An occupational therapist shall determine whether in-person treatment is necessary (this is something that every telehealth practitioner should be doing)
- Connecticut
  - Telehealth does not include fax, voice only calls, texting, or e-mail communication
  - Consent must be obtained during the first telehealth interaction and documented in the patient's medical record. If the consent is revoked, that should also be documented in the chart
  - No facility fee for telehealth services
- Florida
  - Provider may use telehealth for evaluation. If they are able to diagnose and treat the patient with the information obtained from the evaluation, then they are not required to

research the patient's medical history or conduct a physical examination (other states require physicians to complete a physical examination in person prior to a telehealth session)
- A telehealth provider and a patient may be in separate locations when telehealth is used to provide health care services to a patient. In my opinion, this is not specific enough. Does this mean the provider can be on vacation in another state/country?
- Must document that the session occurred via telehealth in the patient's medical record
- Out-of-state telehealth provider registration is available for others to treat Florida residents

- Idaho
  - Provider and patient relationship must be established by two-way audio and visual interaction

- Kentucky
  - Informed consent must be obtained before telehealth services are provided
  - Confidentiality must be maintained (again, something we should all be doing)

- Maryland
  - Cites AOTA Position Paper on Telehealth
- New York
  - Occupational therapist providing services via telehealth must comply with the same standards that apply to in-person practice
- North Carolina
  - Occupational therapist may live in North Carolina without a North Carolina license and treat clients in other states; must follow those state laws
  - Occupational therapist may live in another state and hold a North Carolina license and treat North Carolina residents
- North Dakota
  - Cites AOTA Position Paper on Telehealth
  - The location of the patient at the time of service determines the location of the service. If in North Dakota, occupational therapists must be licensed in North Dakota.
- Oregon
  - Informed consent must be obtained for telehealth prior to the initiation of occupational therapy services

- Secure and maintain confidentiality of medical information in accordance to HIPAA
- Texas
  - Telehealth is the practice of occupational therapy with clients who are located in Texas at the time of services
- Washington
  - Occupational therapists/occupational therapy assistants must be licensed in Washington
  - It must be identified in the clinical record that occupational therapy occurred via telehealth
- Wyoming
  - Consent must be obtained and documentation maintained in the client's health record

The following states have no statute or regulations specific to occupational therapy and telehealth or telemedicine:

- Alabama
- Arizona
- Hawaii
- Indiana
- Maine
- Massachusetts
- Michigan
- Missouri
- Montana
- New Hampshire
- Rhode Island
- South Carolina
- South Dakota
- Tennessee
- Vermont
- West Virginia
- Wisconsin

Please note that this does not imply that we are free to practice across state lines. The general understanding is that you must be licensed in the state where the client resides.

5 EMPLOYMENT

Now you have an idea on how to treat and provide interventions via video. You've done all your research on laws in the state that you're licensed in. What's next? I should have probably put this chapter in the beginning of the book, because many occupational therapists are looking for telehealth job opportunities. When I first launched my telehealth business, more occupational therapists contacted me to inquire about hiring, than clients looking for services.

In no particular order, let's review some of the big telehealth companies that I have come across. If you work or own a telehealth company that employs occupational therapists and I did not mention you in this book, I apologize. Feel free to contact me via email in preparation for the next edition. Okay, moving along. Let's start with

Presence Learning. Dog ear this page or flip your book face down on the table for a second and open up YouTube. Type this: "Telepractice: Your Path to Work/Life Balance". All right, come back…COME BACK!!! Did you get sucked into all the amazing videos they have? If that first video doesn't make you want to become a telehealth provider (otherwise known as telepractitioner), I don't know what will. I'm not here to speak to the quality of the work or employee satisfaction of Presence Learning, but they sure have a great marketing department, don't they?

All humor aside, Presence Learning is a school-based telehealth company providing occupational therapy and speech-language therapy, as well as other special needs services. They require a minimum of two days weekly during typical school days and additional availability for consults and IEP meetings. They use the following online assessment tools: Beery VMI, MVPT-4, Sensory Profile 2, Sensory Processing Measure, and School Function Assessment. Presence Learning uses their own proprietary platform that engages the children on the screen. For the practitioner, it is a one-stop shop for billing, scheduling, and documentation.

Similar to Presence Learning, TalkPath Live provides speech-language therapy, occupational therapy, physical therapy, mental health and behavioral counseling, and early intervention services. TalkPath Live also has proprietary technology and they pride themselves in the use of their technology across difference types of devices. TalkPath Live mentions both occupational therapy and occupational therapy assistant positions and the support they provide to their service providers. What I found most interesting about this company is that they serve both children and adults. They contract with schools, healthcare facilities, and individuals.

In contrast, TinyEYE Therapy Services is dedicated to online speech and occupational therapy for schools only. TinyEYE also has proprietary software with online activities for the students and therapists to use, but the most fascinating thing about this company is that they have a robot that they provide to the schools for group learning. They also use an e-helper or an individual who helps the student with the software platform. The platform also includes an online backpack that the therapist can include therapy notes, homework, and other activities to practice at home or at school. The child's progress is monitored between each session.

Therapy Source is another company that provides school-based jobs only. They classify themselves as a staffing company and outline the benefits of working for them as: flexible schedule options, nationwide presence, competitive rates, contract relationship, and much more. Again, Therapy Source uses a proprietary platform called TheraWeb where the therapist and the client can play games or just engage in a simple video call. The Therapy Source website has a couple of great examples of occupational therapy telehealth sessions using the TheraWeb platform. They also have an interesting concept of a blended approach to therapy, combining in-person and online sessions for school-based services. They are using telehealth services to fill in the gaps in missed sessions due to illness, school closure, and other absences.

  DotCom Therapy is another telehealth company. I remember first hearing about them a long time ago and, looking at their website now, it looks like they have expanded their services a lot. They are providing schools with audiologists, case managers, mental health providers, occupational therapists, and speech therapists. They also provide a private client program that starts at $49 per week and caters to both children and adults. From an employee perspective, what stands out the most about DotCom Therapy is that they hire W-2 employees; provide health and dental insurance, a 401k, and other benefits. I know many occupational therapists are looking for work in telehealth, but do not want to settle for independent contractor (1099) status. Therefore, DotCom Therapy is a great option for employment from that standpoint.

The last telehealth company that I want to discuss is Global Teletherapy. Global Teletherapy, like Therapy Source, is a staffing company that is providing occupational therapists, speech-language pathologists, and mental health counselors to schools nationwide. Some of the benefits of working for Global Teletherapy include flexible schedules, free access to assessments and resources, and a competitive pay rate with 25% extra for documentation and prep time. They do have a 10-hour per week minimum and encourage occupational therapists to get licensed across multiple states to build a caseload quickly. They also mention that they provide occupational therapists and the clients with a tool kit of familiar objects used in school-based interventions; including scissors, putty, pompoms, handwriting sheets, crayons, and more. The purpose of this is so that the occupational therapist and client can easily interact with the same items.

I have provided a brief overview of six telehealth companies, but trust me when I say that there are many more to choose from. My advice is to do your research and make sure you do not sign anything that says that you cannot work for another telehealth company. I have heard of colleagues working for multiple companies, rather than seeking additional state licenses, as this can be pricey. Another piece of advise is to ask the telehealth company that you are applying for to pay the state licensing fees if they want you to be cross-licensed.

6 REFERRALS AND PAYMENT SOURCE

Referrals

If you've gotten this far in the book, you're probably much more interested in starting a private practice rather than just working for one of the big telehealth companies. If this is the path that you are setting out on, then the next question is probably, "Where do I get referrals?"

When I first got into private practice and I asked this question, the most popular answer I got was, "Word of mouth." Being the over-analytical person that I am, that just left me wondering where did the very *first* client come from. How exactly did word of mouth get started? After learning a lot about marketing, I finally understand that sales and marketing is about building relationships. I am, by no means, a marketing expert, but my number one tip to get clients is to start talking to people. Tell everyone about your practice even before you get your business license. Keeping in mind that you have to start building relationships with all types of people, let's go over some of the more structured ways to get referrals. I will keep this section very brief, because you should probably go read a whole different book on marketing in private practice after you finish with this book.

The first person that comes to mind when we think about referrals is a physician. This can be a primary care physician, a neurologist, an orthopedist, or a developmental pediatrician. Any and all of these physicians should know about occupational therapy and should be referring their patients to us. Sadly, the truth is that many physicians don't have the time to meet with us and get to know us well enough to build a relationship with us. However, if you can find the opportunity to build a relationship with a physician, they can be a great referral source. One thing I should note here is that, depending on the state you are practicing in, if you are a cash-based occupational therapist, you may or may not need a prescription from a physician. Of course, you can still build the physician relationships for referrals, but it's nice not having to rely on them for an occupational therapy order. This is known as direct access to services.

In pediatrics, another great referral source is schools. You may find it difficult to get into a public school system as a private practice owner, but private schools are a great avenue to explore. If you find a private school that does not have an occupational therapy program, that could be a gold mine of clients ready for your services. Along the same lines as schools, one strategy that I heard that has a lot of success is doing daycare screens. Providing the teacher or parents with a simple developmental checklist, and completing a child observation in the room, can offer more than enough information to make a recommendation for an occupational therapy evaluation.

Another great source for referrals, believe it or not, is other occupational therapy private practice owners. If you read the acknowledgements in the beginning of this book, you know that I am extremely grateful for the one occupational therapist that let me observe her telehealth sessions. Sadly, others saw me as a threat to their company and were not willing to share information with the "competition". Keep in mind that I was a student at the time and not an entrepreneur. I tell you this, because I want to emphasize the importance of camaraderie within our field. There is absolutely no need to feel threatened by one another, especially in the telehealth arena. Think about how many individuals we can serve in one given state; way more potential clients than practitioners.

The last referral source that I want to mention is organizational groups. Often, organizations that support a specific diagnosis have a list of providers to share with families. Getting your name on a list of recommended providers is a great way to obtain referrals. Keep in mind that just having your name on the list is not going to be as effective as building a relationship with a representative from that organization. Fill your calendar with video calls, with various types of individuals, as a way to market yourself. Before you know it, you won't have so many empty spaces in your calendar and you will have a waitlist of clients.

Payment Source and Billing

"Do you take my insurance?" is probably one of the most frequently asked questions in my private practice. Unfortunately, this can be a very complicated question with a complicated answer. Like my professors used to say in occupational therapy school, "It depends." That is not really the answer that I give potential clients, but it is the answer to the question, "Does insurance cover telehealth services?"

The long explanation is that it varies by state. There is something called a parity law, which means that telehealth must be reimbursed at the same rate as in-person visits. However, not every state follows this law. Actually, 28 states mandate parity for Medicaid reimbursement and only 16 states mandate parity for private payers. Even though this sounds like a huge step in the right direction, it is important to note that many states still do not even include occupational therapy in their statutes.

It is my understanding that some private payers are reimbursing for telehealth occupational therapy services. I highly recommend contacting each payer to determine rates of reimbursement for telehealth. To bill commercial insurance, a code modifier of 95 should be used. As for Medicare, unfortunately, occupational therapy is not included in the covered telehealth services. Medicare only covers services provided by physicians, nurse practitioners, physician assistants, clinical nurse specialists, clinical psychologists, clinical social workers, and registered dieticians or nutrition professionals. As mentioned earlier, Medicaid reimbursement varies by state. Please refer to the Center for Connect Health Policy's State Telehealth Laws and Reimbursement Policies document for further information.

From my experience, most telehealth providers that are serving individuals are considered cash-based. Those that are serving schools are under contracts that use the academic budget. There is one more option that is great for private practitioners and that is the use of government scholarships for reimbursement. In Florida, the Gardiner Scholarship provides funds for families of children with autism spectrum disorder and other diagnoses. These funds are for children that do not attend public school and can be used to pay for private school tuition, tutoring, and specialized services including occupational therapy. I do not know whether this or a similar option is available in every state, but I do know, from talking to other colleagues, that Arizona, New Mexico, and California have student scholarships that are used to pay for occupational therapy. This is an option that is worth looking into for those setting out into private practice.

Whether you are trying to launch a private practice, because you have an entrepreneurial spirit, or you want to start exploring telehealth jobs for more flexibility, by reading this book, you have already put your foot one step into the future. The best advice that I can give you is to enjoy the process of becoming a telehealth practitioner!

REFERENCES

Cotton, Z., Russell, T., Johnston, V., & Legge, J. (2017). Training therapists to perform Pre-Employment Functional Assessments: A telerehabilitation approach. *Work, 57*(4), 475–482. https://doi-org.ezproxylocal.library.nova.edu/10.3233/WOR-172578

Gately, M. E., Trudeau, S. A., & Moo, L. R. (2020). Feasibility of Telehealth-Delivered Home Safety Evaluations for Caregivers of Clients With Dementia. *OTJR: Occupation, Participation & Health, 40*(1), 42–49. https://doi-org.ezproxylocal.library.nova.edu/10.1177/1539449219859935

Latour, D. (2019). Unlimbited Wellness: Telehealth for Adults with Upper-Limb Difference. *Journal of Prosthetics & Orthotics (JPO), 31*(4), 246–256. https://doi-org.ezproxylocal.library.nova.edu/10.1097/jpo.0000000000000263

Little, L. M., Pope, E., Wallisch, A., & Dunn, W. (2018). Occupation-based coaching by means of telehealth for families of young children with autism spectrum disorder. *American Journal of Occupational Therapy, 72,* 7202205020. https://doi.org/10.5014/ajot.2018.024786

RESOURCES

http://info.tinyeye.com/

https://doxy.me

https://globalteletherapy.com/

https://txsource.com/

https://vsee.com

https://www.aota.org

https://www.blinksession.com

https://www.cchpca.org/about/national-telehealth-resource-center-partners

https://www.dotcomtherapy.com

https://www.hhs.gov/hipaa/index.html

https://www.nota-app.com

https://www.parinc.com

https://www.pearsonassessments.com

https://www.presencelearning.com/

https://www.simplepractice.com

https://www.talkpathlive.com/

https://www.telehealthresourcecenter.org/

https://www.theranest.com

https://www.theraplatform.com

https://www.wpspublishing.com

https://www.zoom.us

*This book is not sponsored by any of the companies listed in the Resources section.

ABOUT THE AUTHOR

Dr. Reina M. Olivera has been an occupational therapist for 6 years. During that time, she tired to remain a generalist, practicing in almost every setting and population, although her heart has always been in pediatrics. She wanted to be a pediatrician since three years old, but fortunately life lead her in the path of occupational therapy. She obtained her Masters of Occupational Therapy from Nova Southeastern University in 2013 and went directly on to the Doctorate of Occupational Therapy program. She finished her studies at Nova Southeastern University in 2017. While in the doctoral program, she worked in an outpatient pediatric clinic and saw a need to improve parent carryover in the home environment. That is when she learned about telehealth. She has always had a love for technology; therefore, telehealth was a great fit. Dr. Olivera wrote her capstone paper on the use of telehealth in the home environment for families of children with autism spectrum disorder. Now, she runs her own private telehealth practice specializing in working with children with autism spectrum disorder who are homeschooled. She also does online courses on telehealth for other occupational therapists and consulting for those wanting to add telehealth to their private practice. Dr. Olivera can be reached directly at info@telehealthotservices.com or (954) 501-0707.

Made in the USA
San Bernardino, CA
18 March 2020